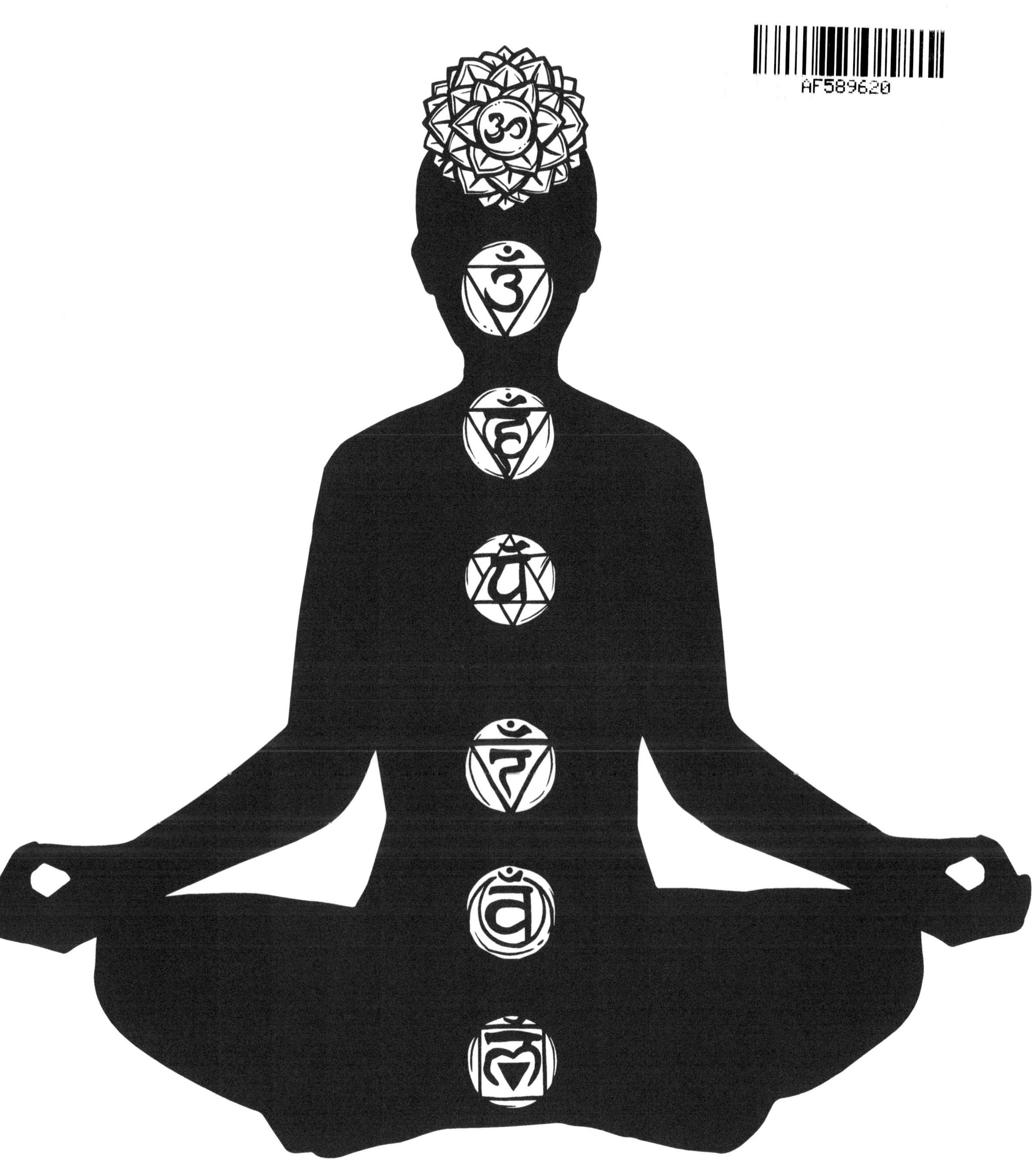

YOUR SUBTLE BODY: UNDERSTANDING THE KOŚAS AND THE CHAKRA SYSTEM

MICHELLE RIGHETTI

CYA E-RYT 500, REIKI MASTER TEACHER, TAO HANDS PRACTITIONER

THE INFORMATION IN THIS BOOK HAS BEEN CAREFULLY RESEARCHED, COMPILED, AND PASSED DOWN THROUGH THE ORAL TRADITION OF YOGA, AND COMPLEMENTARY MODALITIES AND ACCORDING TO OUR BEST KNOWLEDGE AND CONSCIENCE. THE INFORMATION IN THIS BOOK IS MEANT TO BE USED FOR THE EDUCATION AND PRACTICE OF THOSE INTERESTED IN YOGA. THE PRACTICES AND INFORMATION IN THIS BOOK ARE NOT A SUBSTITUTE FOR ANY QUALIFIED MEDICAL ADVICE OF A PHYSICIAN, NATUROPATH, OR OTHER QUALIFIED MEDICAL PROFESSIONAL. THESE PRACTICES ARE MEANT TO SUPPORT THE HEALING PROCESS AND AS AN ADDITION TO, AND NOT AS A REPLACEMENT OF, MEDICAL TREATMENT.

ISBN 978-1-66715-938-6

CLAIRVIDA 233 CARLAW AVENUE, SUITE 816, TORONTO, ON, CANADA, M4M 3N6 WWW.CLAIRVIDA.COM

ORDERING INFORMATION: QUANTITY SALES. SPECIAL DISCOUNTS ARE AVAILABLE ON QUANTITY PURCHASES BY CORPORATIONS, ASSOCIATIONS, AND OTHERS. FOR DETAILS, CONTACT THE PUBLISHER AT THE ADDRESS ABOVE. ORDERS BY CANADIAN AND U.S. TRADE BOOKSTORES AND WHOLESALERS, PLEASE CONTACT THE DISTRIBUTORS: CLAIRVIDA OR VISIT CLAIRVIDA.COM

RIGHETTI, MICHELLE. YOUR SUBTLE BODY: UNDERSTANDING THE KOŚAS AND THE CHAKRA SYSTEM / MICHELLE RIGHETTI .P. CM.

YOGA—HEALTH & WELLNESS - FITNESS - SPIRITUALITY - SELF-HELP - YOGA - MEDITATION - CHAKRAS

This book is dedicated to my yoga teachers: Olga Righetti, Beatrix Montanile, Alanna Kaivalya, Nicki Irwin, Todd Wolfenberg.

Your generous spirits and welcoming hearts paved the pathway for me to discover my calling as a yoga teacher. Your wisdom and understanding opened the doors for the gifts of yoga to make a difference in my life. And In teaching others how to hold this space for this journey, I am reminded constantly of your courage, your love, and your wisdom. Thank you for making this possible, and for sharing your gifts with me.

May you receive their blessings many times over. Namaste.

About The Author

Michelle Righetti is a Reiki Master Teacher, certified e-500 RYT Yoga Teacher, and the cournder of Clairvida, a 1000 Hr Gold-RYS. She comes to this practice from her work as an Actor, Singer, Dancer and Director, and following over a decade of service in the airline industry. Michelle holds her honours B.A. in Music and Culture and Drama at the University of Toronto. She has since studied Applied Linguistics at York University, completed her Reiki Master Teacher Certification, 200 hr Yoga Teacher Training Certification, TEFL-TESOL Language Teaching Certification, and Tao Hands Practitioner Certification.

After experiencing serious injury, Michelle discovered that Reiki, Yoga, and Meditation allowed her to heal her body and opened an entirely new dimension to her creativity.

Now, she teaches and mentors others in these practices so that you, too, can unleash this freedom and healing power.

Clairvida offers professional training, workshops and classes in Reiki, Yoga, and related modalities for adults and children.

About Yoga

This course is designed to provide an in-depth understanding of the seven major chakras, as described in the Hatha Yoga Pradipika, Yoga practice, and related modalities. Chakras are represented as wheels of energy in the body, and blockages in your own chakras (or the restriction of the flow of energy in those areas) can show up as lingering emotions, tension, pain, restriction or repeated experiences that leave you frustrated and stuck in a loop.

Our aim is to help you understand the human body from the perspective of this energetic system. That this may help you to come back into balance, or approach your yoga practice with an awareness of this dimension of our existence. And, to become a stronger, more conscientious teacher of yoga with this knowledge.

Table of Contents

Welcome

Welcome to Understanding the Chakras! This course will help you to understand the koshas, or layers of the body, and how these layers interact with the Chakras, or wheels of concentrated energy that can be found in the body.

This book is an accompaniment to the training of the same name, which comprises of a 6 hour, Continuing Education accredited course, intended to be completed independently or as part of your 200 Hour Yoga Teacher Training, and includes a written test and practicum.

All students are welcome, and invited to learn, participate, and apply this knowledge to your understanding of the human body, and to further your understanding of the yoga practice.

An Introduction to The Subtle Body

The right will I will speak,
and I will speak the true,
May That (Brahman) protect me; may That
protect the teacher.
Om! Peace! Peace! Peace!

—Taittiriya Upanishad,
Translated by Swami Sharvananda

The Taittirīya Upaniṣad is a sacred Vedic text, which is contained as three chapters within the Yajurveda, meaning "yajur=worship and veda= knowledge). The Yajurveda is a text that contains instructions, knowledge and practices for use in rituals, by priests, and in ceremonies, and this is a veda is further broken down into two books: The Krishna (generally known as the "dark" Yajur, as in non-illuminated or mysterious), and the Shukla Yajurveda (generally known as the "bright" or illuminated).

The Krishna Yajurveda has four surviving recensions, or supplementary texts, of which the Taittirīya Upaniṣad is the most well-known.

Here, the sage Tittiri explores the Atman (Self, Soul), and asserts that knowing one's Self/Soul is the path towards liberation from fears, concerns, and to welcoming a blissful state of being. This concept is echoed in the psychological concept included in Maslow's Hierarchy of Needs. The upper-most tier is self-actualization/self-realization, which includes knowing or understanding the Self, so as to achieve one's full potential, including expression through creative activities.

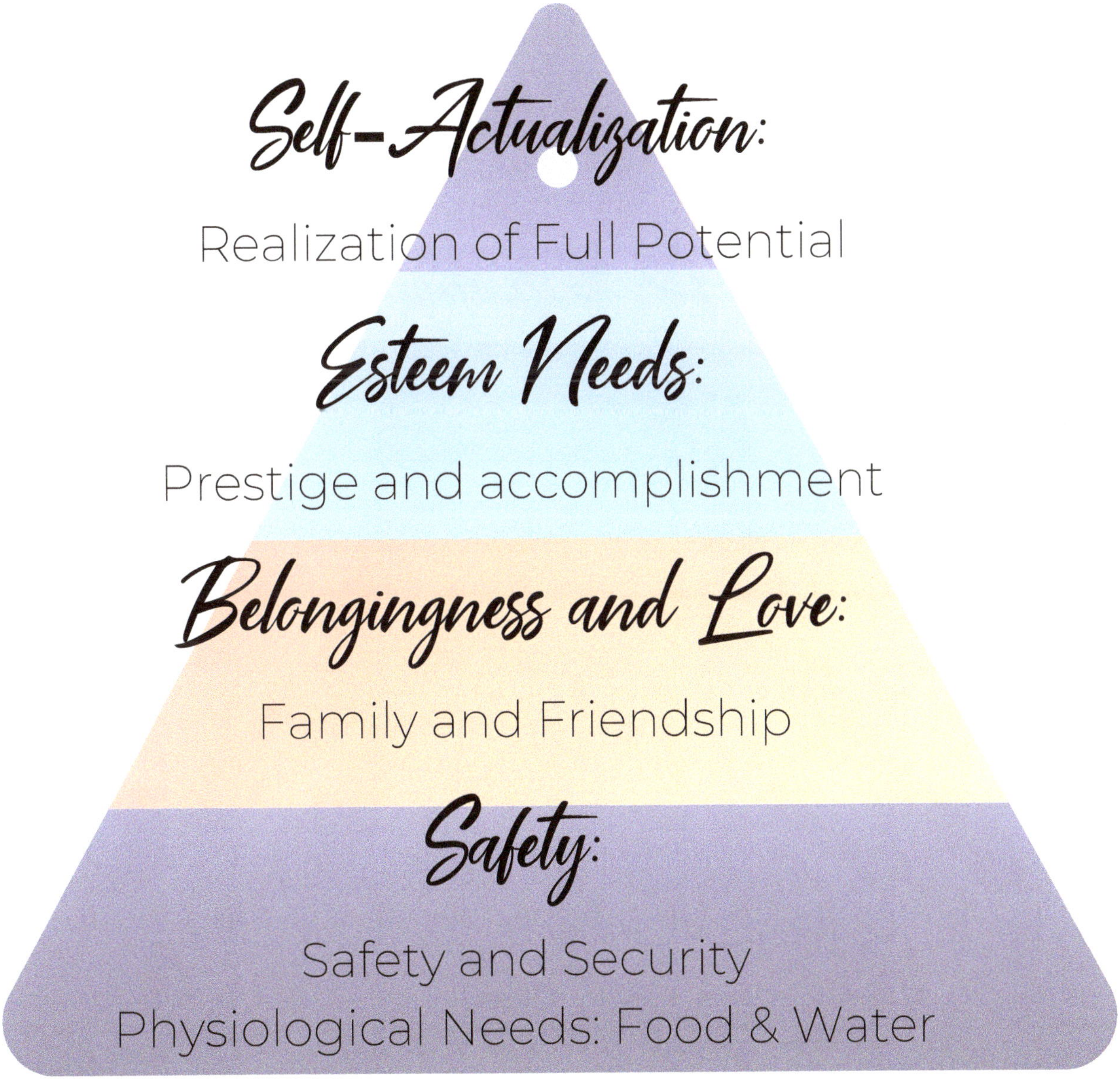

Self-Actualization:

Realization of Full Potential

Esteem Needs:

Prestige and accomplishment

Belongingness and Love:

Family and Friendship

Safety:

Safety and Security

Physiological Needs: Food & Water

-Maslow's Hierarchy of Needs

Layers of The Subtle Body

According to Tittiri, the Atman (Self) can be broken down into five layers, called Kośas (pronounced Koshas), that might be imagined like the layers of an onion, or are often depicted as a series of Russian Nesting Dolls, one contained within the next.

In chapter 4 of The Taittirīya Upaniṣad, named the Brahmananda Valli, we are introduced to these Kośas.

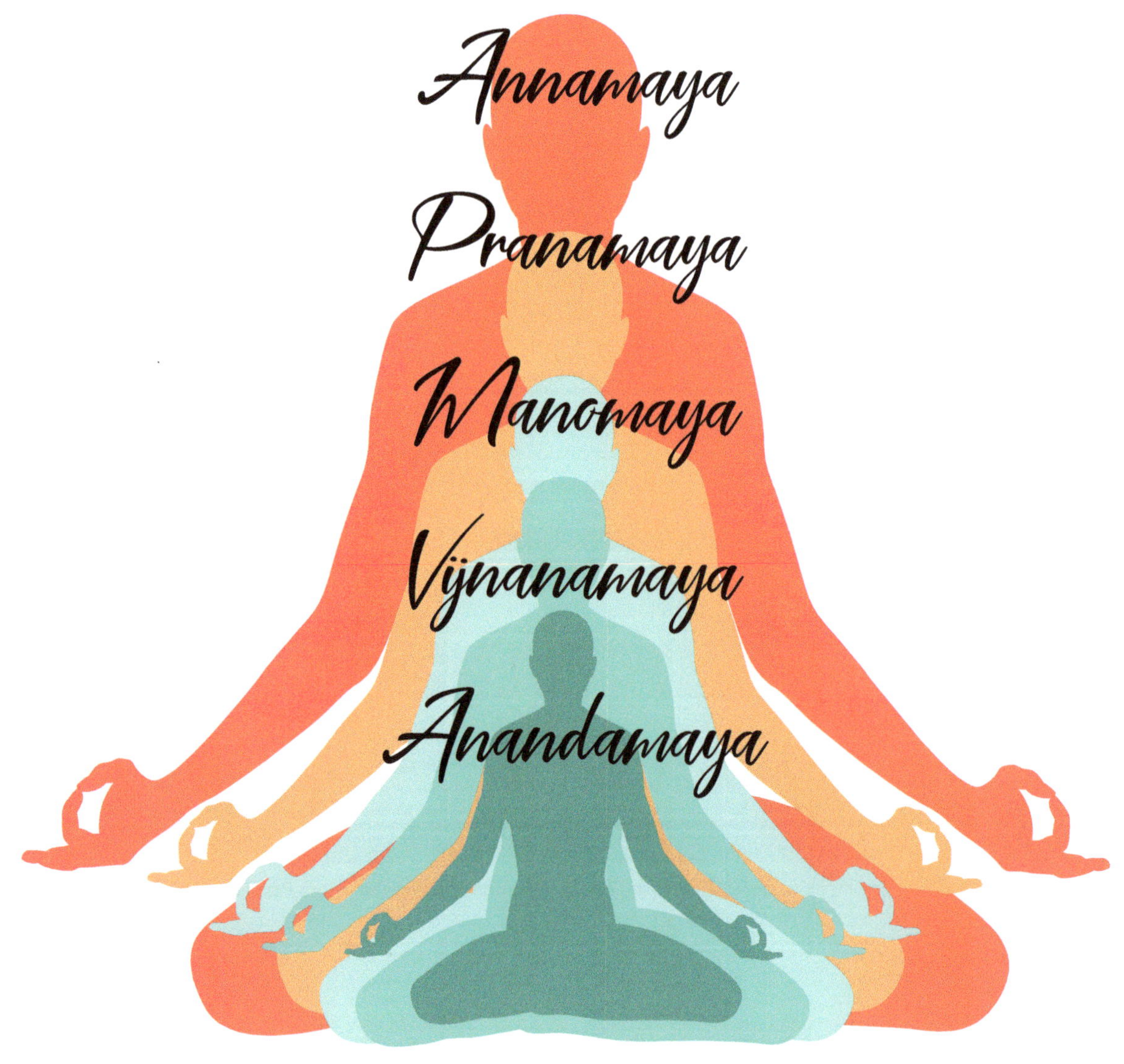

The 5 Kośas

Annamaya Kośa - The Physical Body, or our outermost shell. This is in particular as it applies to our relationship with nature and food, nutrition, and the natural elements.
Pranamaya Kośa- The Energetic/Pranic Body, or the life-force layer. This is related to the way in which we bring energy in and out of the body through pranayama, breathing.
Manomaya Kośa - The mental/emotional body that relates to manas (thought, will, wish), and the concept that it is with the power of thought and will that one determines one's actions, and leads to bliss.
Vijñãnamaya Kośa - The Knowledge/Wisdom body. Nestled within our mind, it contains the knowledge and wisdom associated with ethics, truth, understanding, and achieving a state of yoga, or union of consciousness between one's Atman and Brahman states.
Anandamaya Kośa - the Bliss layer. Through the wisdom that comes from understanding all of our Kośas, we arrive at bliss, or the liberation that comes from attaining a state of yoga. And, while this layer is always within us, and part of us, we must constantly nourish and seek to understand all layers so as to continually reach this center within ourselves.

Prana

In Sanskrit texts dating as far as 3000 years ago, such as in the Shiva Samhita (author unknown), the energy, or prana, of the subtle and causal body is said to flow through pathways or lines called Nāḍī.

In other texts and practices, such as in traditional Chinese Medicine, these lines are called meridians. In some depictions, there are hundreds, or even thousands of lines of energy that flo wthrough the body.

If we follow the pathway of *all* forms of energy that move through the body, we can begin to understand the pathways that are taken by our breath, our circulatory system, our nervous system, our endocrine system, our digestive system, our reproductive system, as well as our emotions, our thoughts, movement (kinetic energy), force (such as the movement of force through our skeletal system and out to the Earth or objects which we touch), thermal energy (heat and cold), etc.

Simply stated, Prana is life-force energy. Many ancient texts, from the 3000-year old Chandogya Upaniṣad, to the Mahabarata all reference the prana as containing multiple layers or sources, or ways in which prana moves through the body.

The channels through which prana travels through the body are called the Nāḍīs. The Brhadaranyaka Upanishad (2.I.19) mentions that there are 72,000 Nadis in the human body. Although there are thousands of channels throughout the body, there are only three major or principal Nāḍīs through which the flow of prana can be detected most easily. The three main Nāḍīs are Sushumna, the central Nāḍī , Ida, the Nāḍī originating in the left gonad (testes or ovary), and which spirals upward through the body; and pingala, originating in the right gonad and spiraling upwards in the body.

Prana moves through the body in the form of Vayu, or winds, and can be categorized as follows:

Prāṇa - The the energy of the heart. Moves in the form of emotions, laughter, sorrow, crying, talking, singing, dancing, fighting, actions (karma) and artistic expression.
Apāna- The downward moving energy, or releasing energy. This energy flows in the form of excrement, urination, menstrual blood, and vaginal and seminal fluid.
Udāna - The upward moving energy, centered around the throat. Moves through sneezing, hiccuping, vomiting, coughing, burping.
Samāna- The energy of the navel. Associated with nutrition and our ancestors. This energy mixes with anything that is consumed, such as food or drink, and moves into the body that way (such as nutrition from our food).

Vyāna- The energy of the joints. Moves in the form of goosebumps, sweat, and the movement of joints and of energy through the fascia. (synovial fluid, hyaluronic acid, water, fat, etc.)

The Nāḍīs

The Nāḍīs can be used as a map for perceiving this movement within the human body. If we look at the busiest channels, we can see that there are three main channels through which the majority of energy travels.

Ida - Beginning in the left side of the body (gonads). The feminine, representing the receptivity to energy, inhalation, the moon and lunar cycle.
Pingala - Beginning in the right side of the body (gonads)The masculine, representing action or sending of energy, exhalation, the sun and solar cycle.
Sushumna - The center, representing the balance between all forms of energy in our bodies, the cerebrospinal column, and the pathway the consciousness or soul takes within the body.

You might find it helpful to think of these Nāḍīs as a double helix, centered around a central column of light. This provides us with the imagery contained in the Caduceus symbol, internationally used in representing the practice of medicine.

At the intersection of each Nāḍī, an increase of energy can be seen within the body. Just like a roundabout road, the traffic flows from multiple directions around each roundabout, so while it all flows together, there is naturally an increase in traffic at the intersection. Those intersections in the body are known as the Chakras, and they work together to form the Chakra System.

Using this roundabout as a model, you may imagine this as a circular motion in which all three Nāḍīs co-exist in the same space, increasing the available energy in that spot. Or, you might find it helpful to think of it as light. Where there is one ray of light, there is 30% illumination. However, whenever three rays of light come together, the illumination in that area rises to 90%.

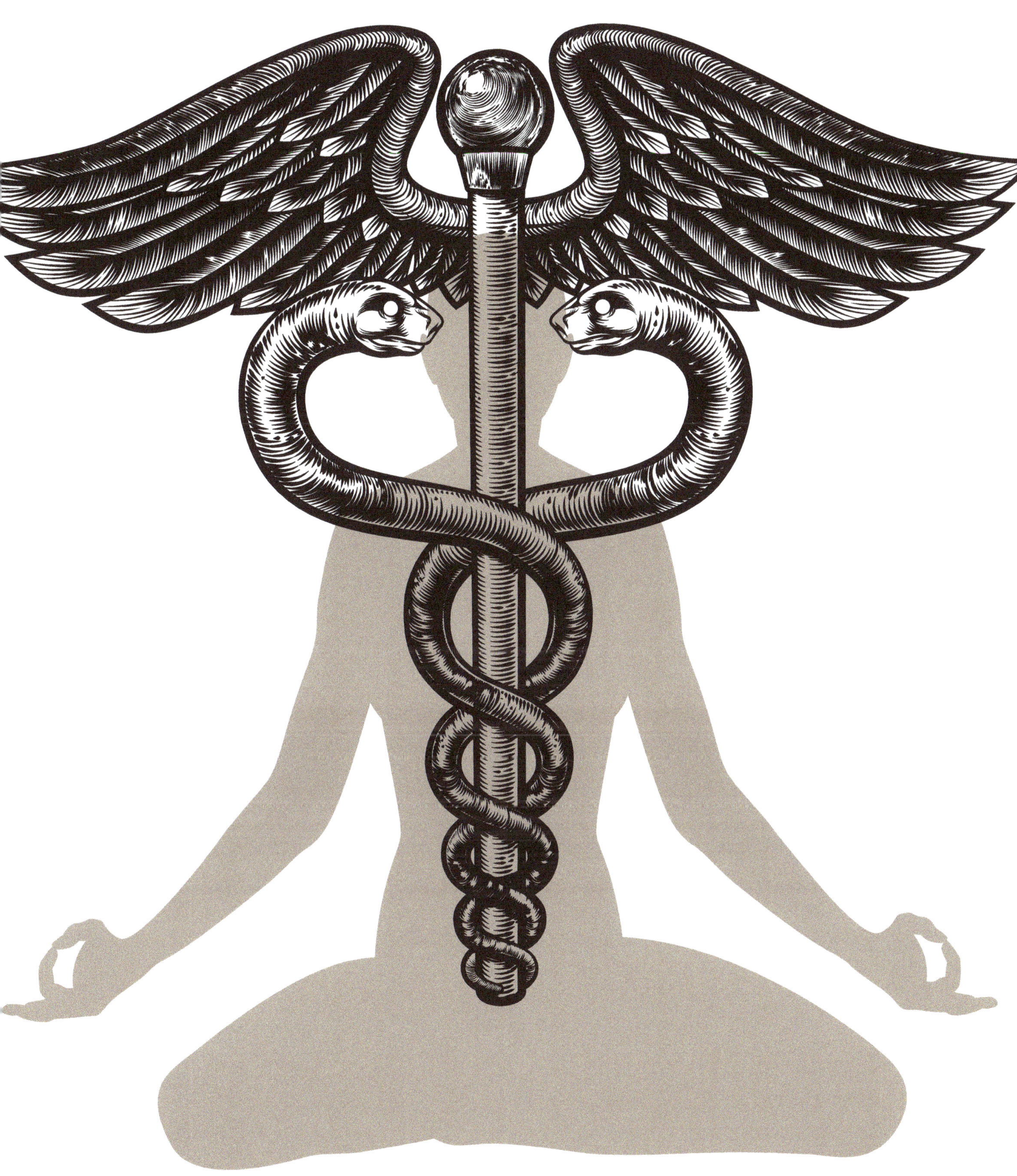

-Caduceus symbol, internationally used in representing the practice of medicine.

The 7 Chakras

While there are perhaps thousands of chakras in the body, there are 7 main Chakras, or principal areas of focus within the energetic body.

Yoga, as well as many other Eastern modalities and practices, share the use of the Chakra System as a map of the subtle body. When we experience pain, tension, or other symptoms in our bodies, it indicates that in that area of the body there is an energetic blockage- that is to say, the prana of the body, (whether in the form of air, heat, force, etc.) is in some way restricted or blocked.

In yoga, we aim to release this tension and ease the flow of prana through movement, stretching, pranayama, and through the training of the mind in letting go of the kleshas (obstacles) that hinder us.

In Yoga, this process is facilitated by the practicing of asana, pranayama, as well as the directing of prana using sequencing which helps to direct the prana to the area of focus and to encourage the flow of prana throughout the body, and all of its koshas.

Muladhara, The Root Chakra

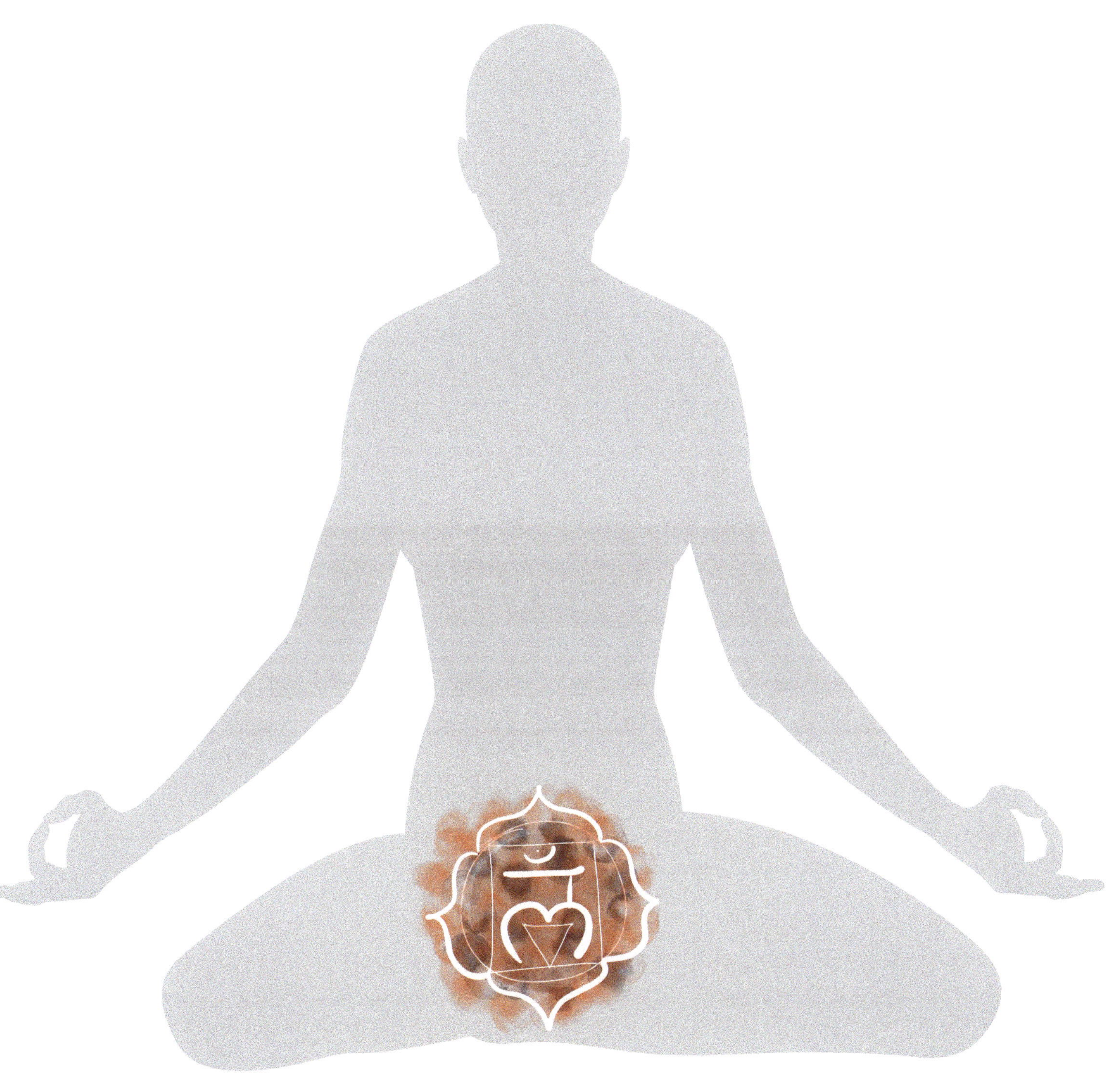

Muladhara, The Root Chakra

Located at the base of the spine, the Root chakra represents the way in which we move through life, and our connection to nature, the present moment, and the yogi's ability to be perfectly at peace at any time. Blockages, such as tension, tightness or pain in this area can be related to the emotions surrounding insecurity, fear, money, stability, home, family, and work.

Symptoms:
Underactive: Depression, low self-esteem, weight loss/gain, immune deficiency,
low sex drive, anaemia, lethargy, procrastination, anxiety, fearfulness.

Balanced: Sense of being grounded, vitality, abundant energy, security, manifesting abundance, mastering one's self, confidence, a sense of self.

Overactive: Egotistical attitude, sexual addiction or overly sexual, materialism,
greed, being easy to anger, impulsive, rigid to change, selfishness, dominating,
controlling, micromanaging.

Bija Mantra: LAM

Asanas: Grounding asanas, standing and balancing asanas, tadasana, trikonasana, padangustasana.

Swadhisthana, The Sacral Chakra

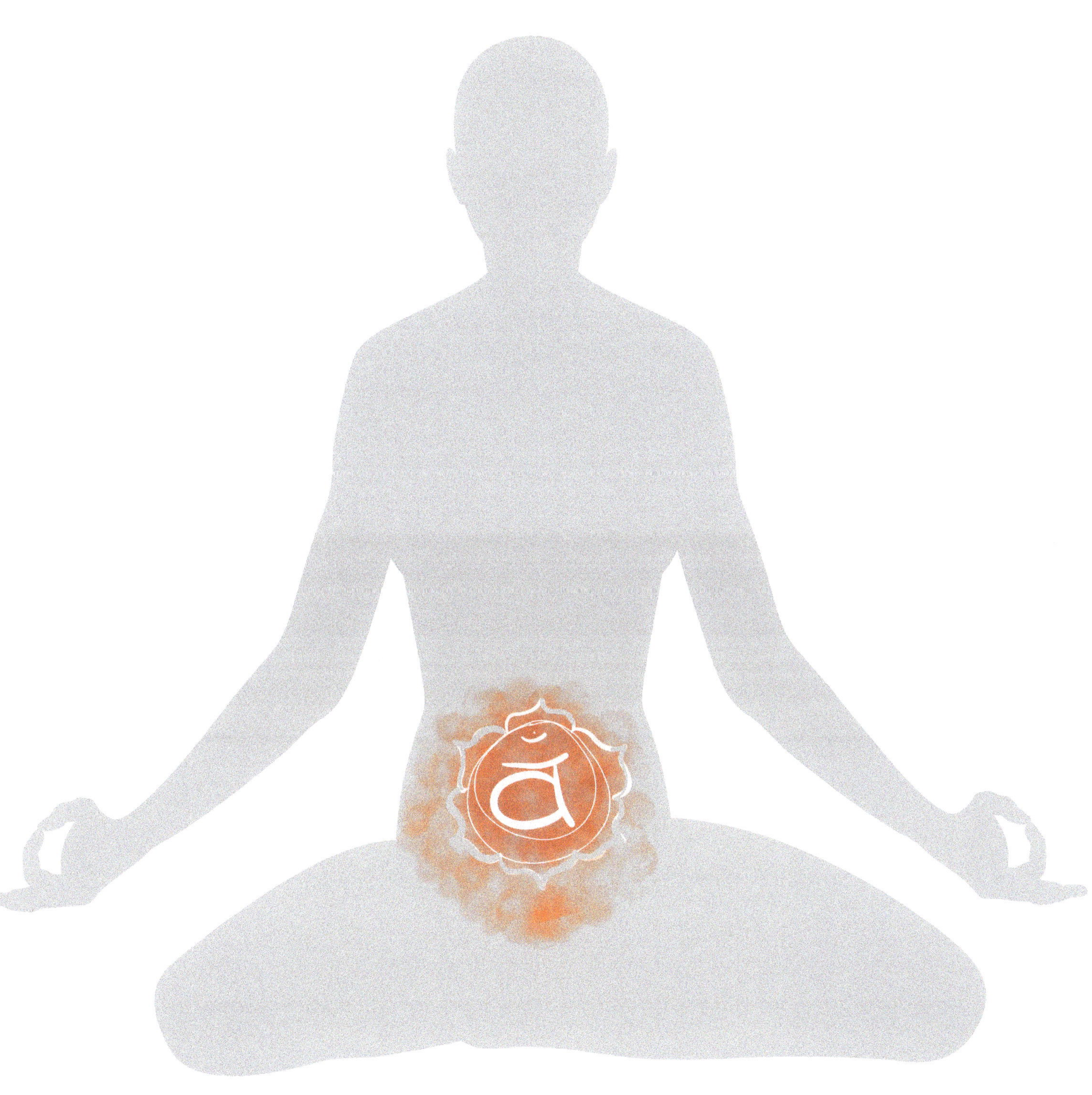

Swadhisthana, The Sacral Chakra

Sanskrit for "dwelling place of the Self ", located just below the navel, and at the level of the sacrum. This Chakra relates to our physical manifestation, creativity, and sexual energy. Blockages in this Chakra can be related to our sense of self-worth, social relationships, and our relationships with others, and how we are manifesting our desires into reality.

Symptoms:
Underactive: Stifled creativity, poor social skills, rigidity, fear of sex or emotional connection, untrusting, lack of passion and excitement, fatigue, fear of change, lower abdominal or lower back pain.

Balanced: Open to intimacy, creativity, comfortable with sex and sexuality, friendly, compassionate, attuned to feelings, graceful movement, experiences pleasure.

Overactive: Addiction to pleasure, self-serving, creates drama, sexual addiction, emotionally sensitive, emotional attachment, manipulation, poor boundaries.

Bija Mantra: VAM

Asanas: Hip openers such as Rajakapotasana, baddha konasana, trikonasana, virabhadrasana III, Ardha Chandrasana, and lower-back and glutes-strengthening backbends such as ustrasana and setu bandha sarvangasana

Manipura, The Solar Plexus Chakra

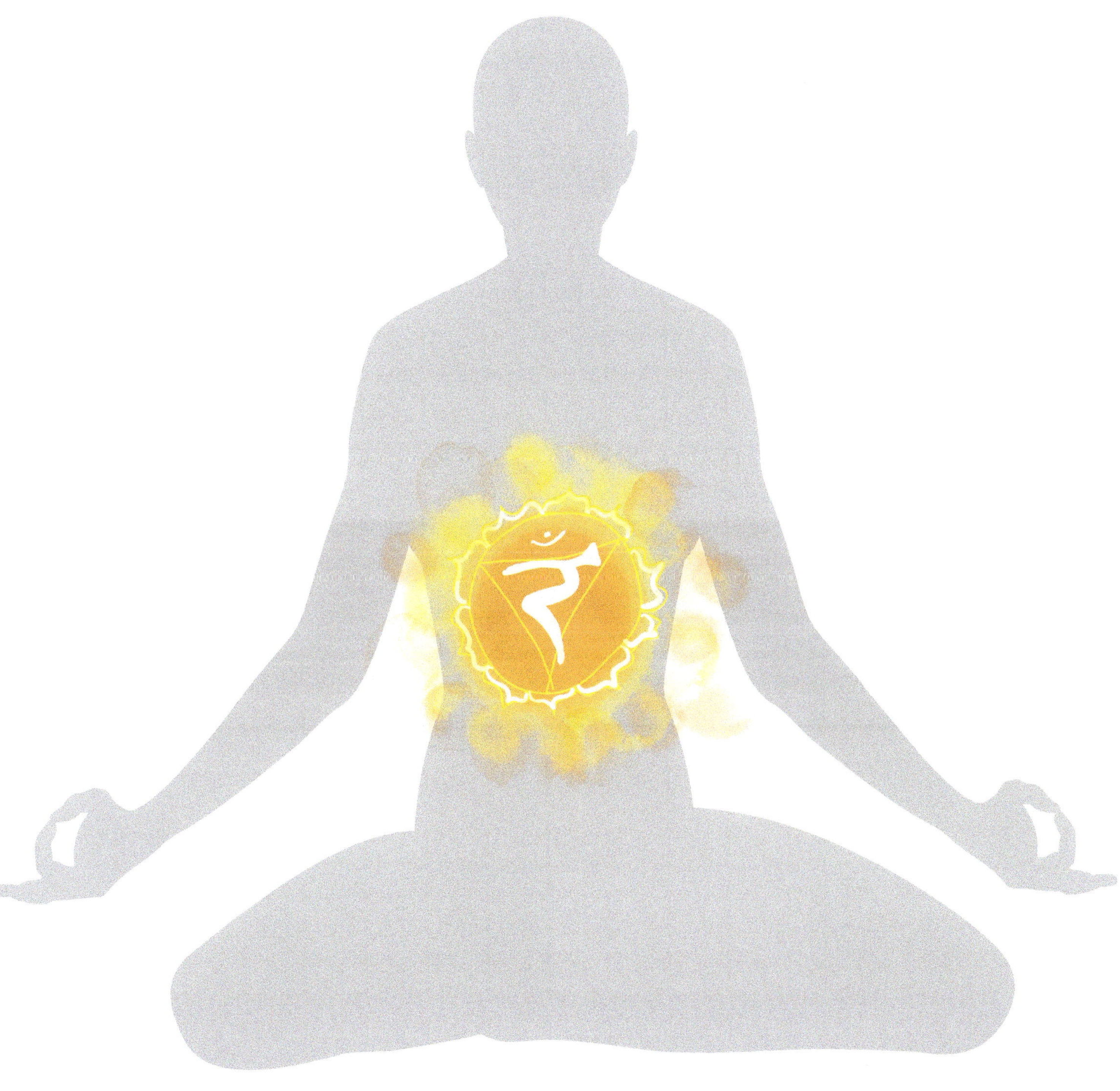

Manipura, The Solar Plexus Chakra

Located above the navel and near the lower ribs, the Solar Plexus Chakra radiates vital energy throughout the body. Wearing clothing that bare the upper abdominal area welcomes the sun to heat and recharges this Chakra. This is the center of the will power, self-awareness, ego and confidence. Blockages, tension or pain in this area can be related to processing of raw emotions and self-discipline, or challenges surrounding personal power, self-worth, clarity and creativity. This is where we gain a mental understanding of our emotional self.

Symptoms:
Underactive: Easily manipulated, blames others, unreliable, poor self-worth,
doubtful, seeking approval, weak will power.

Balanced: Confident, meets challenges, warm personality, knowing without
doubt, responsible, reliable, playful and has a sense of humor.

Overactive: Stubbornness and the need to be right, controlling, aggressive,
manipulative, short tempered, judgmental, planning without action, and
dominating.

Bija Mantra: RAM
Asanas: Practice axial rotation (twists) and backbends to open this chakra, and core strengtheners to provide additional support in this area. Confidence boosters are also great! Try ustrasana, parivrtta parsvakonasana, parivrtta utkatasana, matsyendrasana, and core poses such as phalakasana, navasana, etc.

Anahata, The Heart Chakra

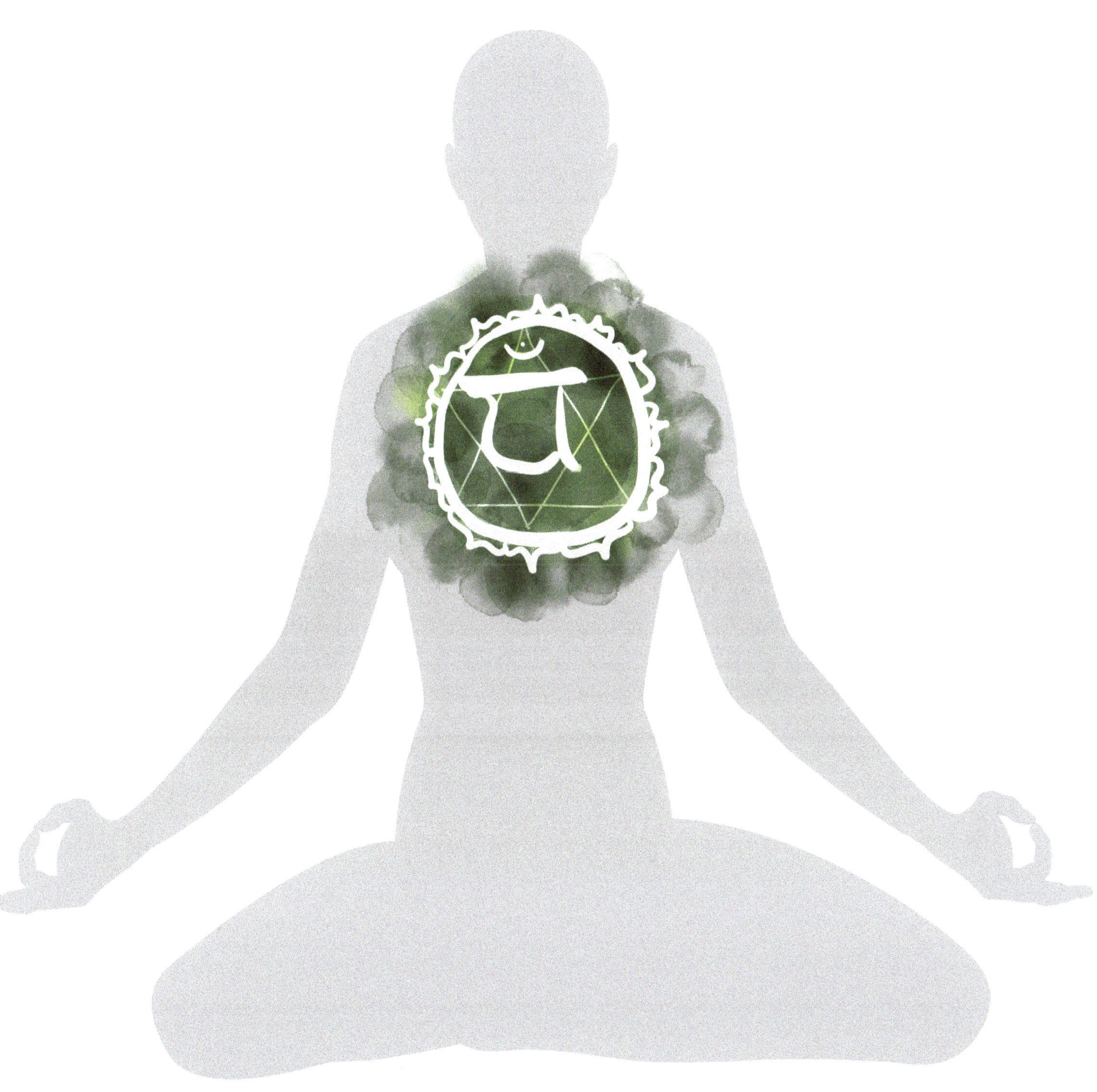

Anahata, The Heart Chakra

The heart is the center of the true self and the Chakra System, and from which love, joy, and compassion all radiate. This Chakra connects the lower Chakras with the higher Chakras. Imbalances in the anahata can be related to emotions surrounding grief, loss, heartbreak, compassion, anger, sadness and love for ourselves and others.

Symptoms:

Underactive: Anti-social, critical, isolated, loneliness, feeling rejected, lack of empathy, negative outlook, feeling unworthy.

Balanced: Joyous, compassionate, understanding, peaceful, loving, connected to all of life, understanding, empathy.

Overactive: Jealousy, clinging, demanding, over-sacrificing, codependency, needs to please, conditional affection or acceptance.

Bija Mantra: YAM

Asanas: To open the heart, practice heart opening asanas, shoulder openers and shoulder strengthening asanas. Try garudasana, uttana shishonasana, camatkarasana, dhanurasana, urdhva dhanurasana or chakrasana, etc.

Visuddha, The Throat Chakra

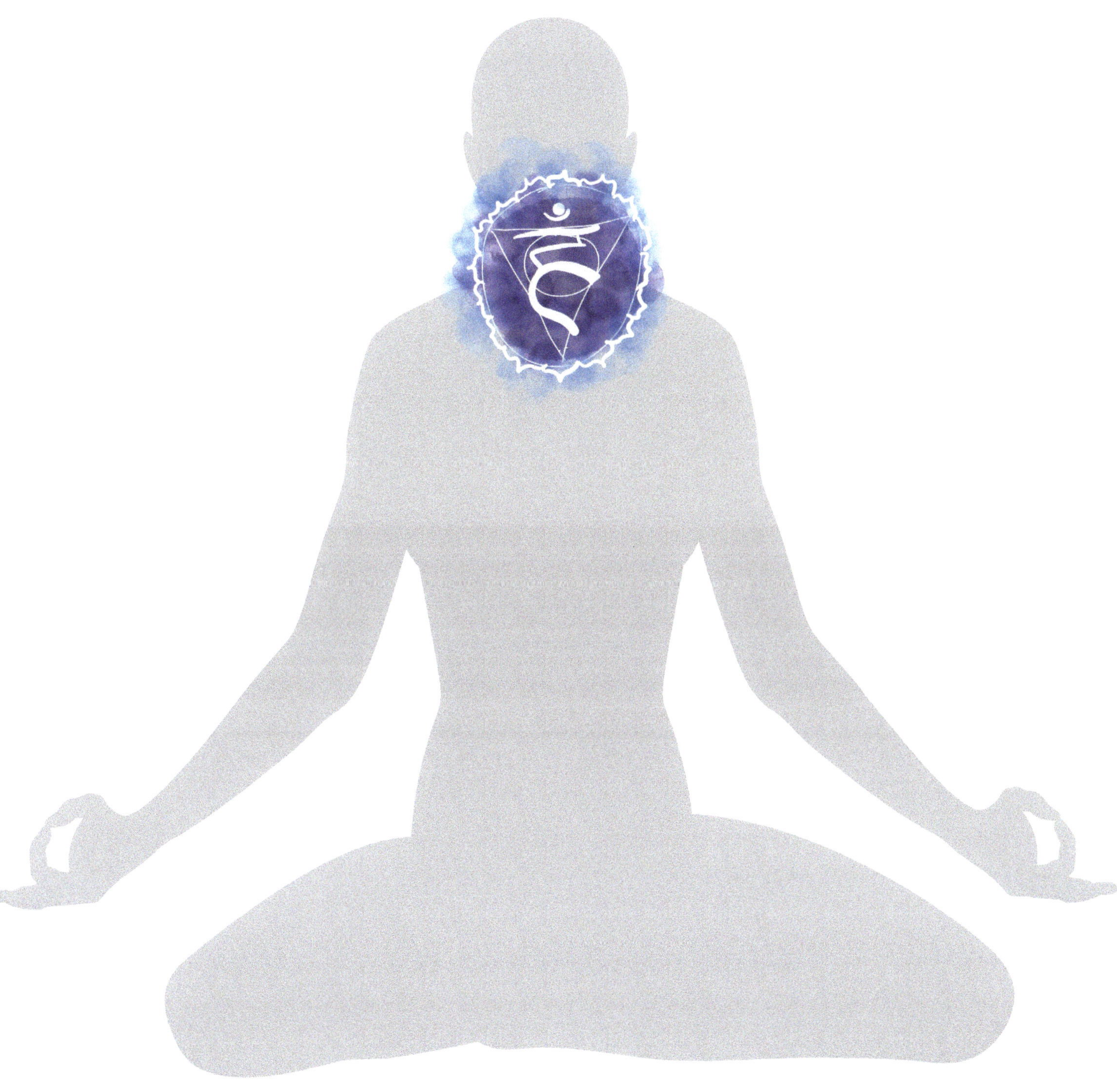

Visuddha, The Throat Chakra

Located at the base of the throat, near the larynx. Blockages in this Chakra can be related to hearing or communicating the truth, or to challenges in seeing things from multiple perspectives. Work on freedom of expression, speaking out Truthfully and with compassion.

Symptoms:

Underactive: Fear of speaking, difficulty expressing thoughts into words, shyness, introversion, withdrawn, out of touch with desires, singing notes are restricted, "vocal fry", flat tones.

Balanced: Expressive of feelings and thoughts, living creatively, fully self-expressed, good sense of timing and rhythm, imaginative, inspired, clear speech.

Overactive: Overly talkative, or unable to censor speech. Defensive or dominating speech or voice, difficulty listening, criticism, overly-opinionated. singing notes are tense, too wide and bright, or sharp tones.

Bija Mantra: HAM

Asanas: Neck stretches, neck rolls and asanas that strengthen and stretch the cervical spine. Trikonasana, Urdhva mukha svanasana, marichyasana, paschimottanasana, simhasana, vajrasana, salamba sarvangasana, chanting, singing, kirtan.

Ajna, The Third Eye Chakra

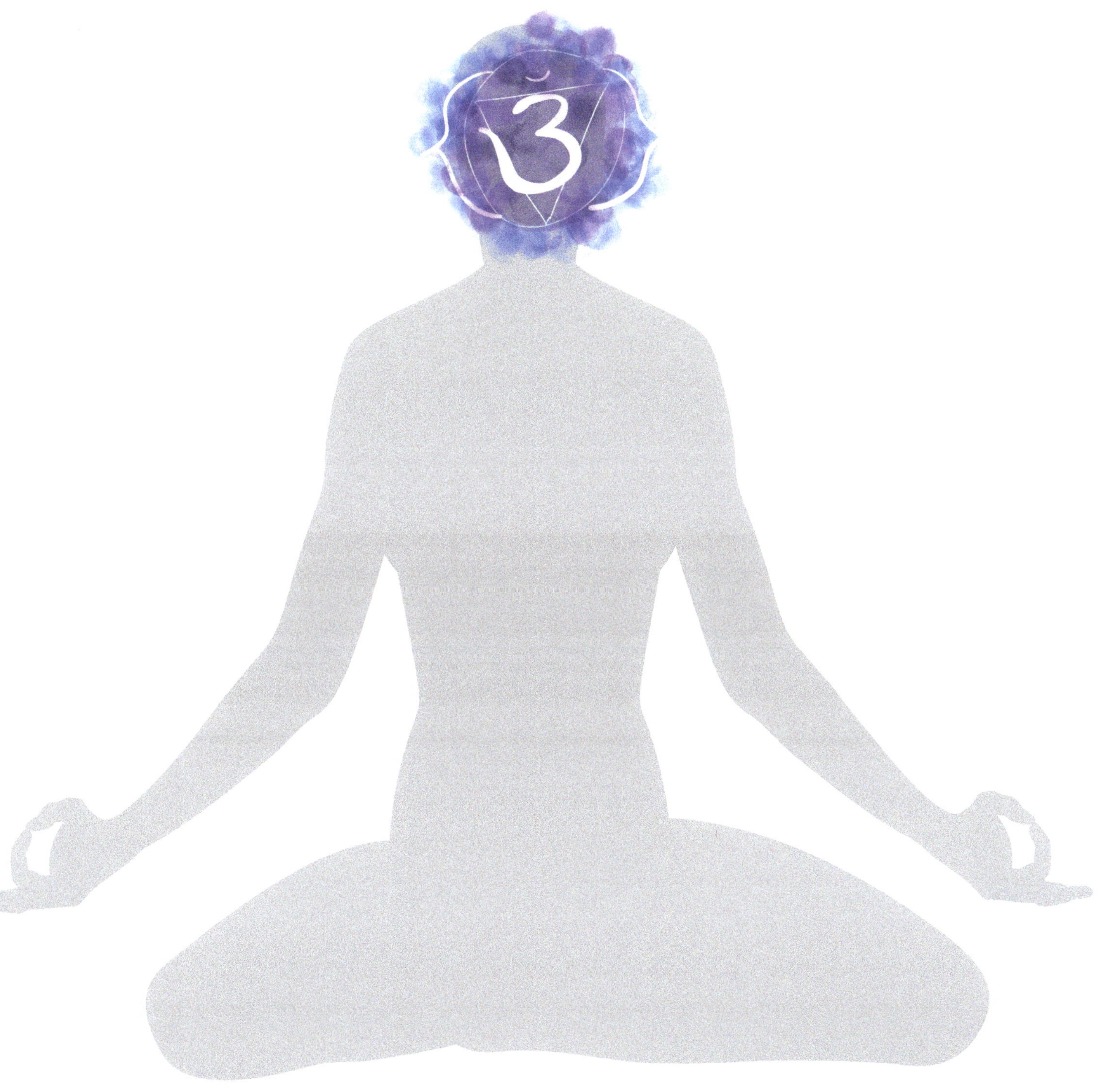

Ajna, The Third Eye Chakra

Located in the center of the brain, behind the centre of the eyebrows. This Chakra is the centre for intuition, mental clarity, dreams, goals and values.

Symptoms:

Underactive: Lack of focus, lack of imagination, difficulty perceiving the future,
poor vision, poor memory, poor common sense, difficulty understanding
inner and outer reality.

Balanced: Intuitive, imaginative, able to experience altered states naturally.
Able to take a step back and look at the world, work through larger ideas, see
through illusion, learn new concepts with ease. Receiving messages from higher
Self, access to the Akashic Records, Spiritual dimensions.

Overactive: Obsessive thoughts, delusion, hallucination, nightmares, stress,
difficulty concentrating.

Bija Mantra: OM

Asanas: Balasana with the forehead on the ground, all pranayama, sirsasana (any variation), sasangasana, chanting, meditation.

Sahasrara, The Crown Chakra

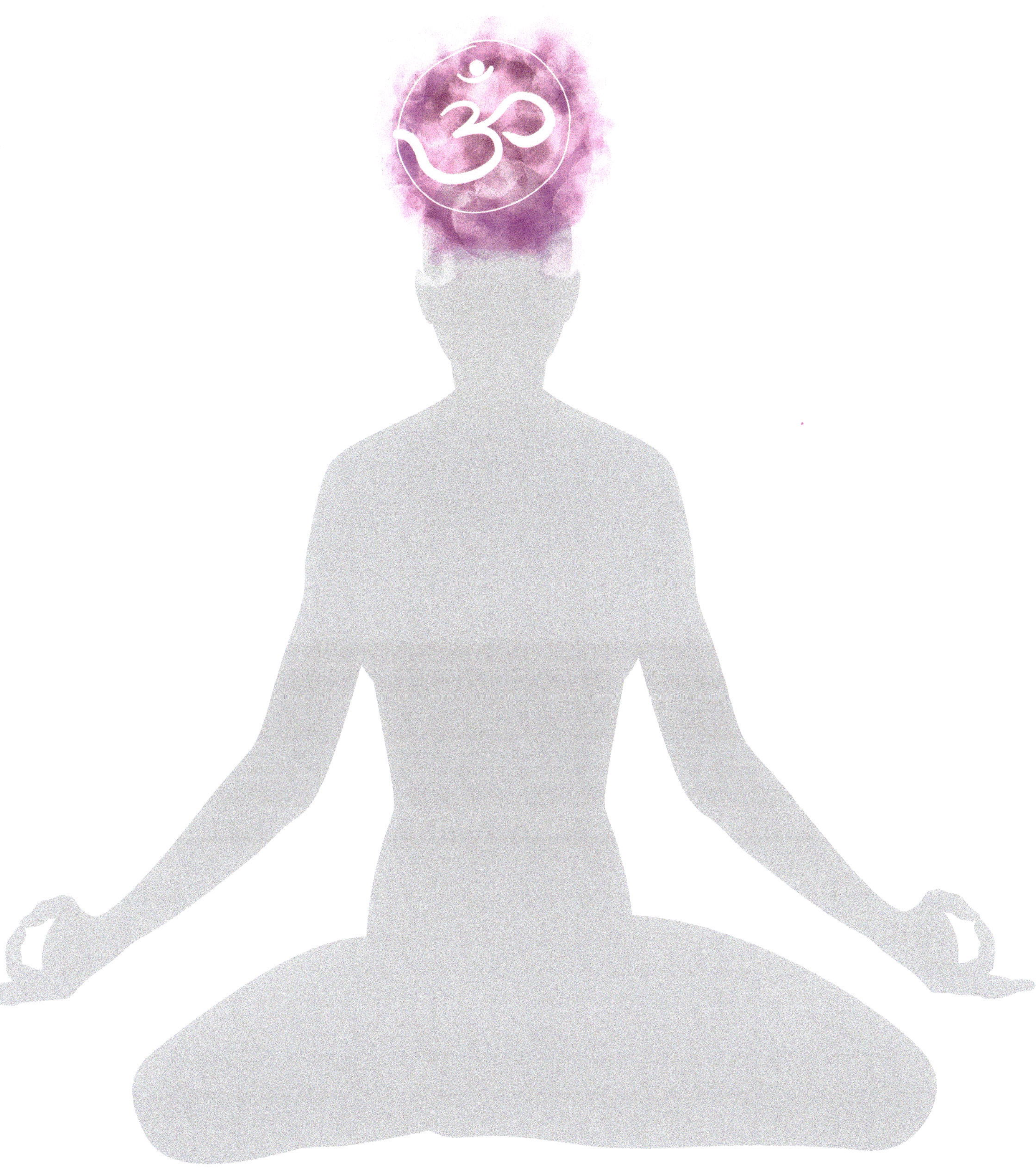

Sahasrara, The Crown Chakra

At the top of the head, the Crown Chakra is our connection with our higher self, the Divine. This portal bridges the physical and non-physical dimensions or layers of our existence. Blockages or tension and pain in the scalp or top of the head can be related to resistance as we become aware of our Divinity, infinite wisdom, and enlightenment.

Symptoms:

Underactive: No zest for life. Lack of joy, melancholy, depression, indecision, lack of purpose, fear of death, no desire to discover inner self.

Balanced: Alchemy, intuitive knowledge, open to divine guidance, miracles, fearless, not fearing death, communion with spirit.

Overactive: Frustration, loss of self, uncontrolled alternate personalities, realm encounters, possession, difficulty grounding, condescending.

Bija Mantra: OM

Asanas: Pranayama, meditation, chanting and kirtan, savasana. Yoga nidra. Bhakti yoga practices. Chakrasana to connect all 7 chakras and open and align the body.

Creating Flow

As you begin to build your yoga classes, you will find that the way in which each pose impacts the energetic body will leave the yogi with a particular feeling or sensation. This is because the way in which asanas stretch, engage, and relax our body impacts the flow of energy through these areas. Think of it as all of the things that move in your body. Circulation, breath, the fluid in our joints, fascia, etc. These are all part of our annamaya kośa- our physical layer. However, the other four kosas are just as impacted by our physical practice. Have you ever rested in a child's pose and found yourself relaxing your neck, only to feel a rush of relaxation move across your shoulders? Or have you relaxed in pigeon pose, feeling the sudden desire to release tears, or sneeze? Or, by contrast, have you ever skipped savasana at the end of class, but found yourself feeling lightheaded, ungrounded or foggy later on? These are all examples of ways in which at times, our many layers show us that they are all intertwined.

As yoga teachers, this provides us with an opportunity to consciously guide our students towards accessing these kośas within themselves, and to possibly let go of some of what no longer serves them, realize that they have been holding onto tension or anger in a place that was unconscious to them, or to discover a source of strength that they didn't realize was possible.

So how do we sequence a class with respect to the chakras and the energetic body?

There are innumerable ways in which a yoga class (specifically a class containing asana practice) can be sequenced. While there is no hard-and-fast rule here, there are some principles which you may find helpful when considering the movement of prana in the subtle body, facilitated through movement.

Think about yoga classes that you have attended. You may recognize the traditional sequence of a 60-minute yoga class as often being something like this:

- Introduction and dharma talk
- Warmup
- Standing asanas
- Balancing asanas, if used
- Forward folds/Backbends
- (or backbends/forward folds)
- Grounded asanas, if used
- Savasana and/or meditation

Take some time to consider the above sequence order, and notice how this impacts the flow of prana. What do you notice? What are some other ways in which you might approach sequencing, and how would your sequence impact the subtle body? Use the following pages to record your thoughts observations, and build your own yoga sequence for the subtle body.

Notes

Afterword

As you begin your teaching journey, you will come to develop your own preferences, experiences, and intuition which will contribute to your unique style as a yoga teacher.

Understanding and bringing awareness to the subtle body can provide access to the ways in which each person holds onto their obstacles, and facilitates a connection with all five kośas.

It is through this awareness of our kośas that we can begin to detect and release the tension and blockages that no longer serve us, and free up our bodies and minds to more easily reach a state of samadhi.

"tatparam purusakhyaterguna vaitrsnyam"

When one has achieved a complete
understanding of their true self,
they will no longer be troubled
by the influences within and without.

-Patanjali's Yoga Sutra 1.16

Thank You

Thank you to everyone who contributed to the writing of this content. To my teachers, my students, and all teachers who came before me. Teaching yoga is one of the greatest gifts.

Thank you also to my partner, my family, and my friends. Your continued love and support provide a pillar upon which I always feel supported as I continue to learn and grow.

And thank you, students. I do not exist as a teacher without you, just as a student cannot learn without a teacher. I am honored and humbled by this gift.

Namaste.

Works Cited

https://www.simplypsychology.org/maslow.html

Desikachar, T.K.V. 1995. The Heart of Yoga: Developing a Personal Practice. Inner Traditions International. 154

Righetti, M. Usui Shiki Ryoho Reiki I: The Essential Guide to a Beginner's Practice. 2020. Lulu Press. 18-27

Tittiri. Translated by Jayaram V. Taittirīya Upaniṣad. 2021. https://www.hinduwebsite.com/taittiriya-upanishad.asp.

www.ingramcontent.com/pod-product-compliance
Ingram Content Group UK Ltd.
Pitfield, Milton Keynes, MK11 3LW, UK
UKHW062010290726
14090UKWH00022B/1485

9 781667 159386